£12.00

T

Surgery for Undescended Testes

General Editor, Wolfe Surgical Atlases:
William F. Walker, DSc, ChM, FRCS (Edin. and
England), FRS (Edin.).

Single Surgical Procedures 11

A Colour Atlas of

Surgery for Undescended Testes

Lewis Spitz

MB, Ch.B, PhD, FRCS(Edin. and England)
Nuffield Professor of Paediatric Surgery, Institute of Child Health,
University of London,
and
Honorary Consultant Paediatric Surgeon,
Hospital for Sick Children,
Great Ormond Street,
London

Wolfe Medical Publications Ltd

Copyright © Lewis Spitz, 1984
Published by Wolfe Medical Publications Ltd, 1984
Printed by Royal Smeets Offset b.v.,
Weert, Netherlands
ISBN 0 7234 1022 4

ISS 0264-8695

This book is one of the titles in the series of
Wolfe Single Surgical Procedures, a series which
will eventually cover some 200 titles.

If you wish to be kept informed of new
additions to the series and receive details of our
other titles, please write to
Wolfe Medical Publications Ltd, Wolfe House,
3 Conway Street, London W1P 6HE

Contents

Acknowledgements

I wish to express my thanks to Mr M. K. Johns, FIMBI, ARPS, Department of Medical Illustration, Hospital for Sick Children, Great Ormond Street, London. It was entirely due to his skill and expertise that all the photography of the procedure was completed in one session. Thanks also to Mrs J. Billington for typing the manuscript and for correcting numerous drafts. Dr A. Filippopoulos prepared the diagrams.

Introduction

Orchidopexy is one of the more common surgical procedures performed on the otherwise healthy male child. Maldescent of the testis occurs in as many as 4.3 per cent of male infants at birth (2.7 per cent for full-term and 21 per cent for premature infants). At six weeks in the full-term and three months in the premature, two-thirds of these testes will have spontaneously descended into the scrotum. The overall incidence of maldescent at one year of age is 0.8 per cent. After this the chances of spontaneous descent of the testis are extremely remote.

Embryology
The gonads develop on the urogenital ridges which are longitudinal structures on the posterior wall of the coelomic cavity on either side of the root of the mesentery of the developing intestine.

Three primordia combine to form the primative gonad:
i)   The primary germ cells, which migrate into the genital ridge;
ii) The mesenchyme of the ventromedial aspects of the mesonephros adjacent to the root of the mesentery;
iii) The coelomic epithelium overlying the mesenchyme. The latter two components together form the genital ridge.

With the arrival of the primative germ cells towards the end of the sixth week of intrauterine life, the epithelial cells covering the gonad grow as cords of cells into the mesenchyme. Between the cords lie the germ cells and gonadal mesenchyme.

Early in the eighth week visible sex differentiation begins. The sex cords continue to develop into seminiferous tubules and rete testis. The tubules of the rete testis become secondarily connected with the mesonephric duct which will eventually form the vas deferens.

Descent of the testis
The stage of so-called internal descent is the result of elongation and differential growth of the posterior abdominal wall structures. During this process, the mesonephros is carried cranially, leaving the testis behind at the level of the internal inguinal ring, where it remains until the seventh month.

True testicular descent begins at 28 weeks and is usually complete at birth. As the testis enters the internal ring, the gubernaculum emerges from the superficial ring. As soon as the gubernaculum reaches the bottom of the scrotum, it begins to contract, drawing the testis caudally. Descent through the inguinal canal takes only a few days, while complete descent into the scrotum is accomplished within the next four weeks.

Failure of testicular descent is likely to be due to either:
i)   A disturbance of the hormonal environment (LH-RH $\rightarrow$ LH $\rightarrow$ testicular hormone axis);
ii) Mechanical failure.

Indications for orchidopexy
1   *Spermatogenesis:* Degenerative changes begin to appear in the undescended testis during the second or third year of life and increase thereafter depending on the duration of the malposition.
2   *Inguinal hernia:* Most undescended testes have an associated patent processus vaginalis. A clinical inguinal hernia is rare but its presence should lead to early surgery to prevent strangulation and/or vascular damage to the testis.
3   *Torsion:* The undescended testis is more prone to torsion because it lies suspended within the patent processus vaginalis.
4   *Trauma:* The undescended testis may be more prone to injury because it lacks the normal cushioning effect of mobility of the testis within the scrotum.
5   *Psychological effects:* It is generally recommended that for psychological reasons it is beneficial to have both testes in the scrotum by the time the child has to attend school.
6   *Malignancy:* There is a significantly increased risk of malignancy developing in the undescended testis (40 times that of the normally descended testis). The risk is greatest for the intra-abdominal testis. Although it has been speculated that early orchidopexy may provide some protection against malignant degeneration, placing the undescended testis in the scrotum clearly facilitates early diagnosis of any subsequent malignant swelling.

Age at orchidopexy
To achieve maximal preservation of spermatogenic function, orchidopexy should be performed around the age of two years.

Diagrammatic representation

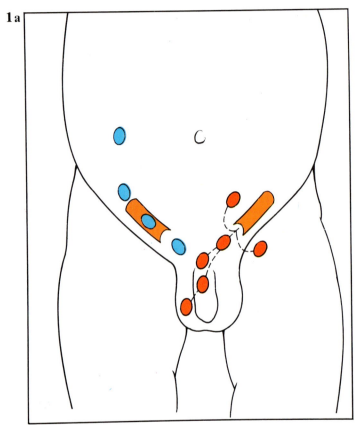

1a

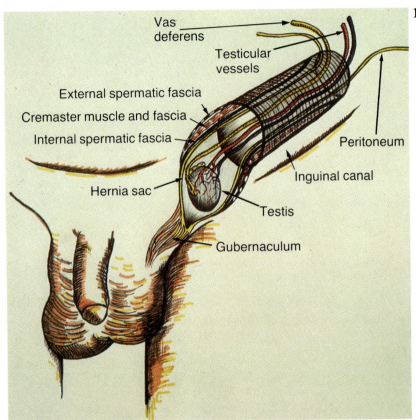

1

Vas deferens

Testicular vessels

External spermatic fascia

Cremaster muscle and fascia

Internal spermatic fascia

Peritoneum

Inguinal canal

Hernia sac

Testis

Gubernaculum

1a Maldescent of the testis. *Retractile testis* is caused by elevation of the testis out of the scrotum and into the inguinal region by the action of the cremaster muscle. It is a normal testis and will return spontaneously into the scrotum when the cremaster muscle relaxes, for example, squatting position, or can be coaxed back into the scrotum by gentle manipulation from the groin.
Ectopic testis is where the testis has emerged through the inguinal canal but has become lodged in an abnormal site, e.g. superficial inguinal pouch, perineum, prepubic, femoral regions (on the left groin in the diagram).

Incompletely descended testis is caused by an arrest of testicular descent along a normal pathway from the site of development in the urogenital ridges of the retroperitoneum to the scrotum (on the right groin in the diagram).

1b Anatomical diagram of the undescended testis. The testis lies just outside the superficial inguinal ring and is associated with a complete hernial sac. The various tissue layers surrounding the testis are shown.

Preparation

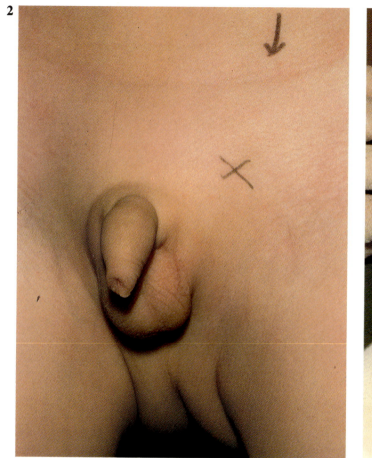

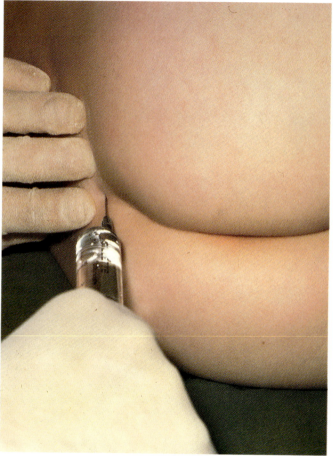

2 Preoperatively the side affected should be marked clearly with an arrow. This will avoid inadvertent surgery on the wrong side. The site at which the testis can be palpated is indicated with a cross.

3 The operation is performed under general anaesthesia. A caudal block may be supplemented to reduce discomfort in the immediate postoperative period. Endotracheal intubation is not usually required, except in the very young infant in whom the operation is being performed primarily for the associated inguinal hernia.

4 **The child lies supine on the operating table with the legs slightly abducted.** A diathermy (electrocautery) pad is applied to the buttocks. Note the identity bracelet on the left wrist. *This is particularly vital in paediatric surgical practice to avoid operating on the wrong patient.*

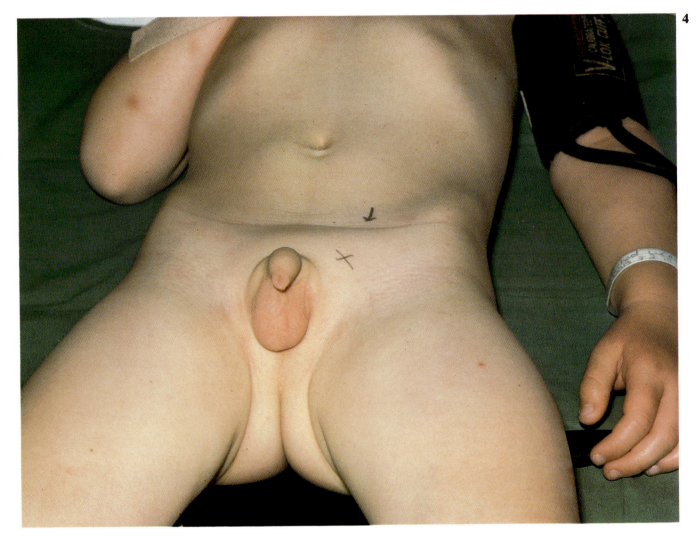

Application of antiseptic and drapes

5 The operative field is prepared by applying an antiseptic solution to the skin over a wide area extending from the umbilicus proximally to the mid-thigh distally. Both groins, the penis, scrotum, and perineum should be included in the prepared area.

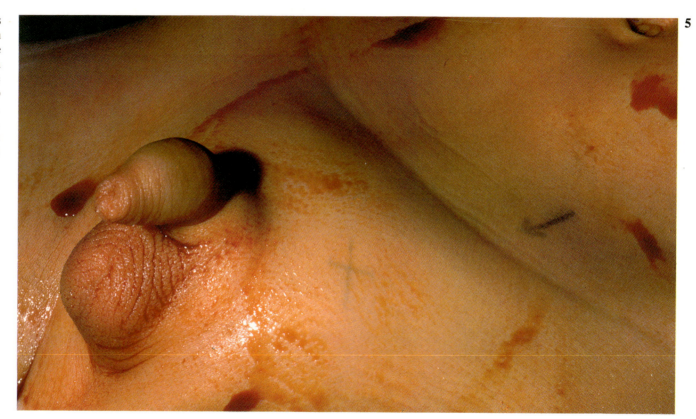

5

6 Sterile drapes are applied leaving the groin on the affected side exposed. The penis and ipsilateral scrotum appear just within the operative field. Note the position of the skin crease in which the incision will be placed.

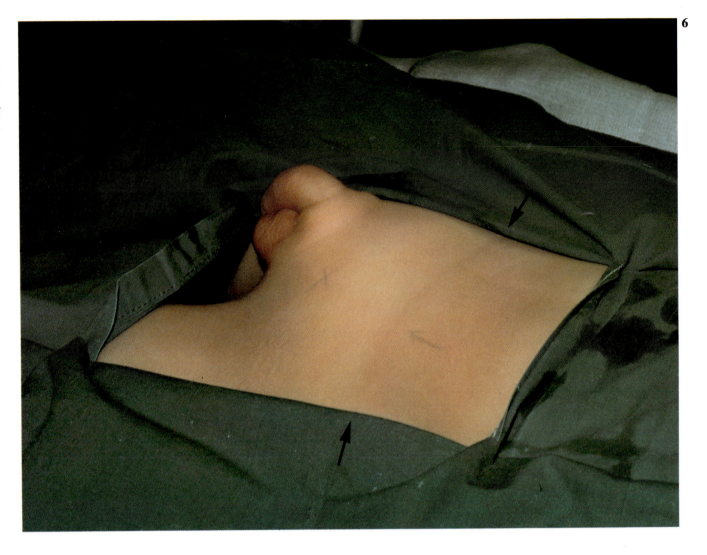

6

Incision

7   The transverse incision is made in the lower-most transverse abdominal skin crease. It extends medially from a point perpendicular to the pubic tubercle to just beyond the level of the mid-inguinal point laterally. The incision is made with a scalpel to the depth of the subcutaneous fat only. The legs of the patient are towards the upper left on this photograph, and the head is on the lower right. Except where stated, all the photographs are orientated from this vantage point.

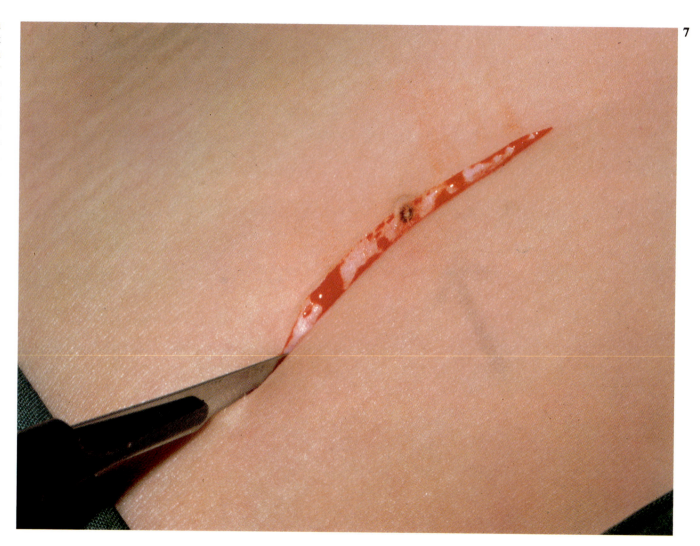

8 To maintain a relatively bloodless operating field, the subcutaneous tissues are divided by means of electrocautery. The cutting current of the diathermy is used for dividing tissue planes while the coagulation current is applied to bleeding vessels to achieve haemostasis.

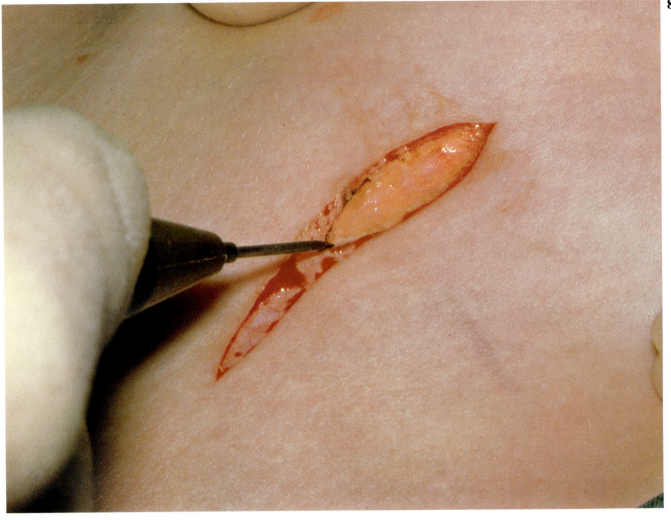

9 The subcutaneous fat has been completely divided, exposing beneath it the fatty layer of Camper's fascia.

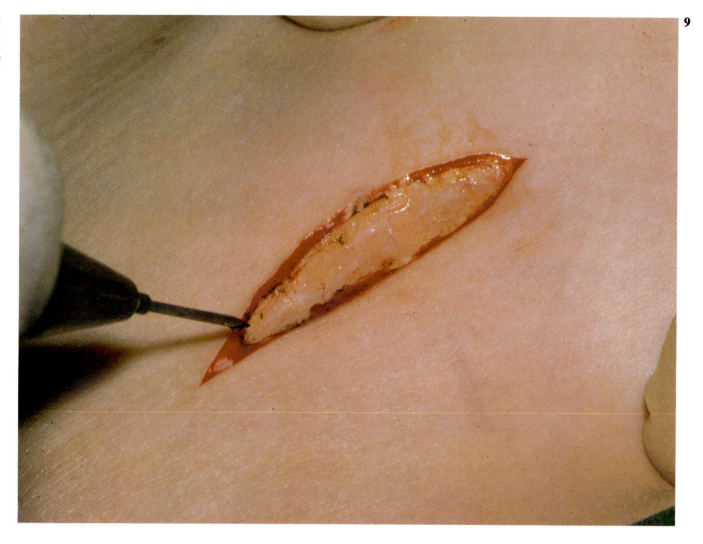

10 The superficial inferior epigastric vein courses across the medial quarter of the incision between the subcutaneous fat and Camper's fascia. This is a constant landmark. Brisk haemorrhage from the wound will occur if this vessel is divided without prior coagulation or ligation.

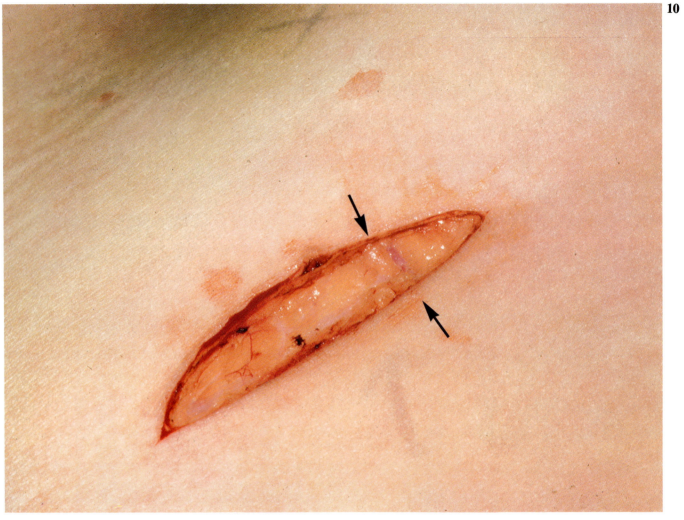

11 A close-up view of the superficial inferior epigastric vein passing across the medial part of the incision. It should be ligated with a fine, i.e. 0000, absorbable material e.g. chromic catgut or polyglycolic acid ligature or cauterized and divided.

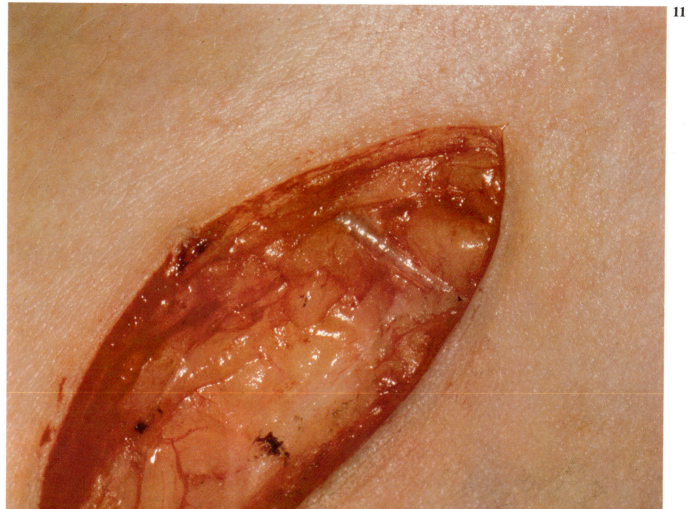

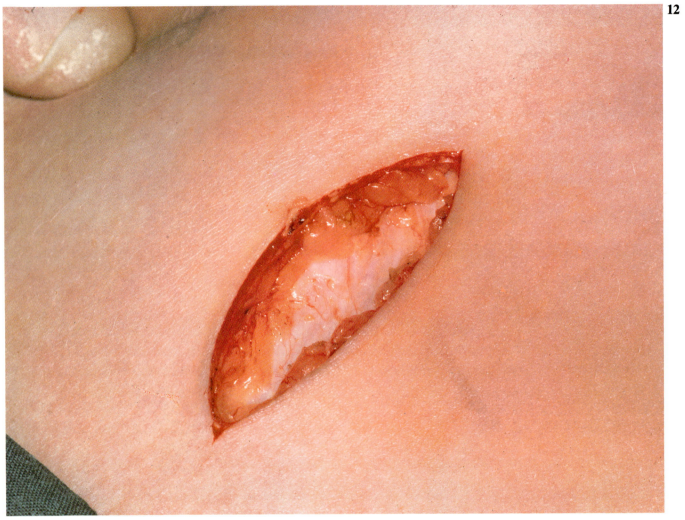

12 The fascia confining the fat of Camper's layer is exposed.

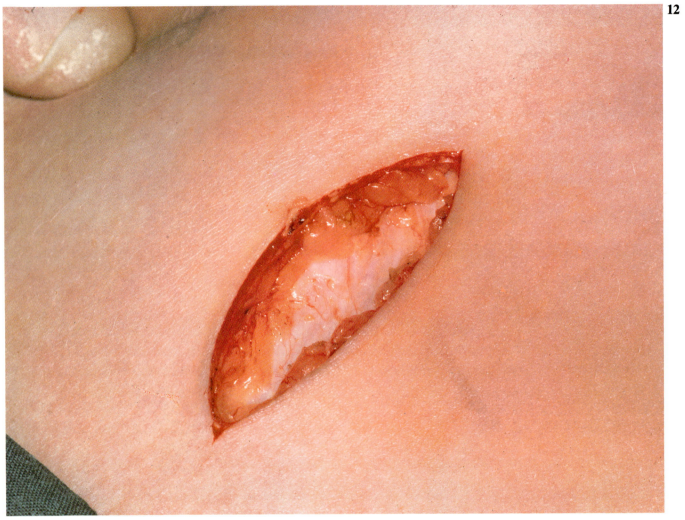

13 **The fascia overlying Camper's layer is grasped between two tissue forceps** and divided using either electrocautery or sharp dissection.

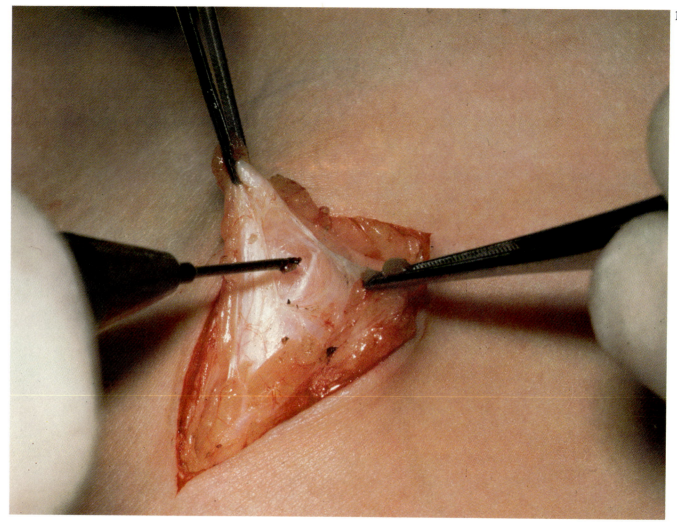

14 **Deep to Camper's fascia lies another well-developed fascial layer, Scarpa's fascia.** In the infant and child this layer is particularly prominent as a separate tissue plane identified by its peculiar grayish-white glistening appearance.

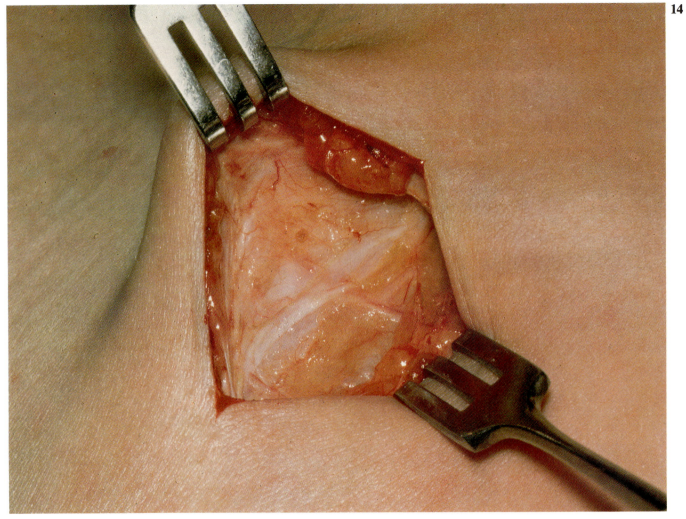

Scarpa's fascia incised and divided

15 Scarpa's fascia is incised and divided throughout the length of the incision.

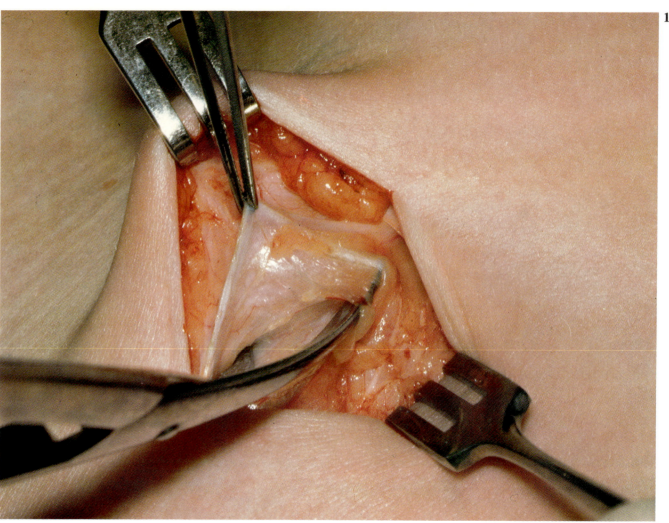

16 Scarpa's fascia has been divided exposing the tendinous fibres of the external oblique aponeurosis which form part of the anterior wall of the inguinal canal. The lowermost fibres of the external oblique aponeurosis are cleared of overlying fascia.

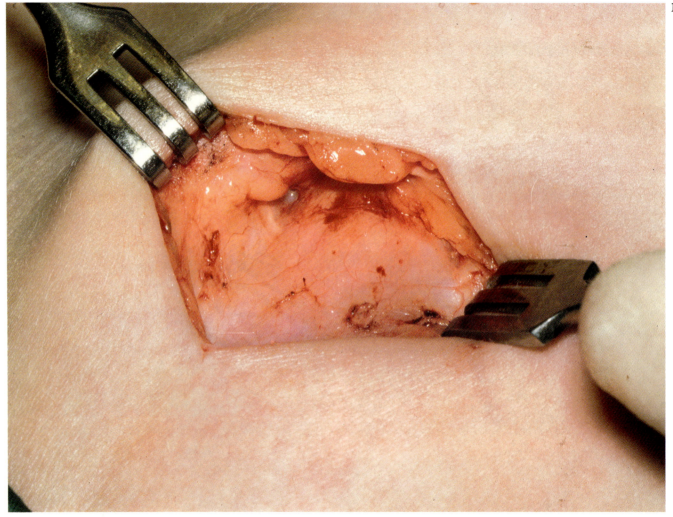

17 Inferomedially, the margins of the oval-shaped external (superficial) inguinal ring are defined. It lies just above and lateral to the pubic tubercle. The spermatic cord passes through the ring and from its margin originates the external spermatic fascia. (When the testis lies within the inguinal canal or intra-abdominally, the external inguinal ring is usually small.)

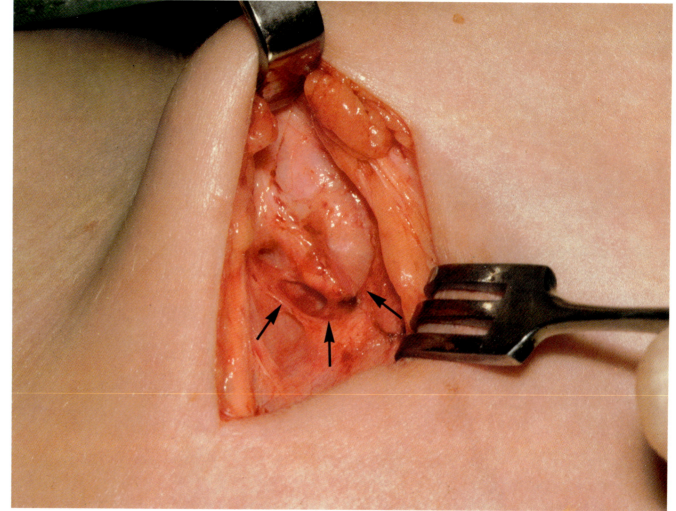

Opening the inguinal canal

18 A short (1 cm), shallow incision is made in the anterior wall of the inguinal canal (i.e. through the fibres of the external oblique aponeurosis) above and lateral to the external inguinal ring. The incision is through the aponeurotic fibres only and should not impinge on the underlying cord.

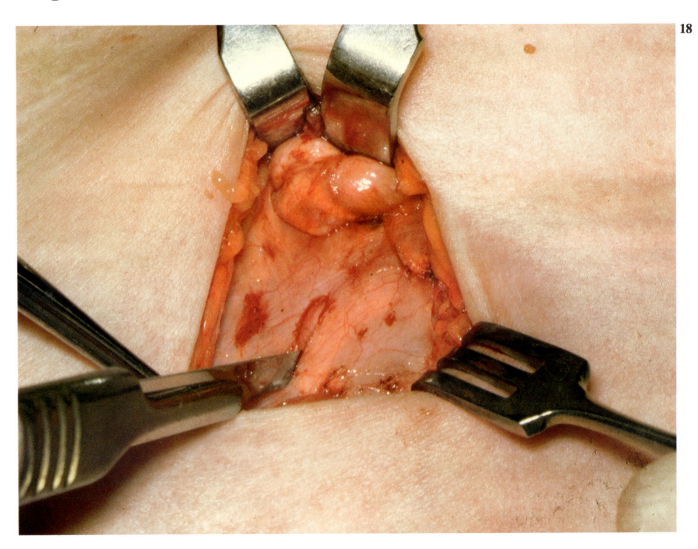

18

19 The edges of the incision in the anterior wall of the inguinal canal are grasped with two fine artery forceps (mosquito clamps).

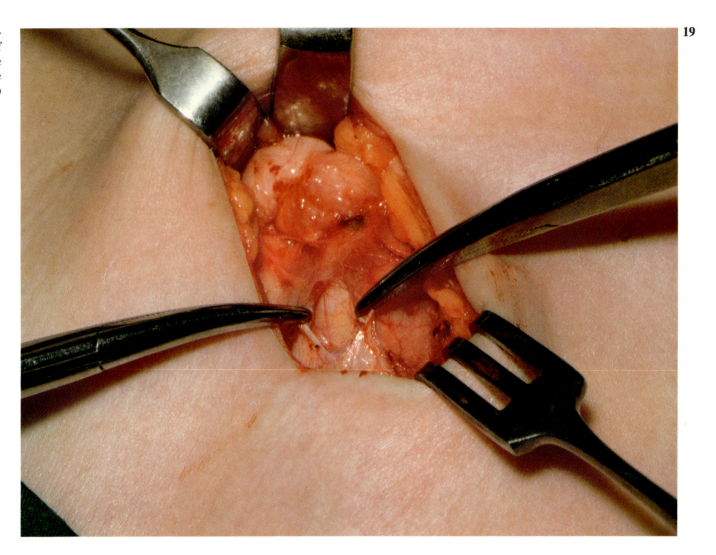

20 The shiny internal spermatic fascia and cremasteric muscle fibres are clearly visible within the inguinal canal. The ileo-inguinal nerve passing on the surface of the spermatic cord towards the external ring should be identified and carefully preserved. It provides the sensory nerve supply to the upper medial portion of the thigh and anterior third of the scrotum.

Division of this nerve results in loss of sensation to the area of supply while damage to the nerve causes uncomfortable paraesthesia.

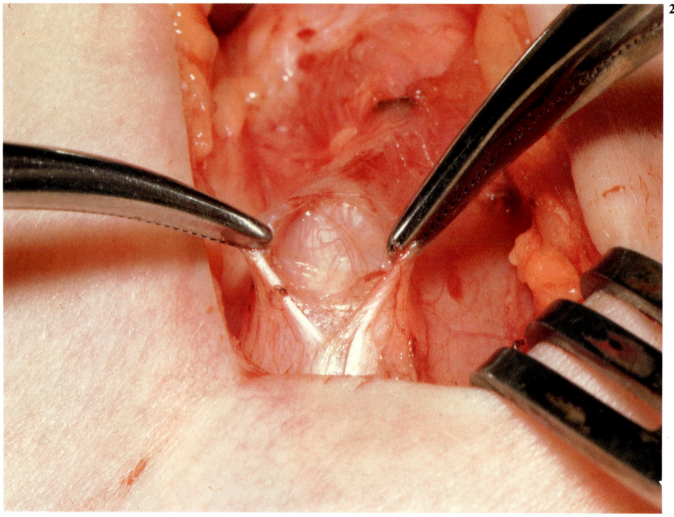

21 The external oblique aponeurosis is mobilised off the surface of the spermatic cord from lateral to medial, until the tip of the scissors emerges through the external inguinal ring.

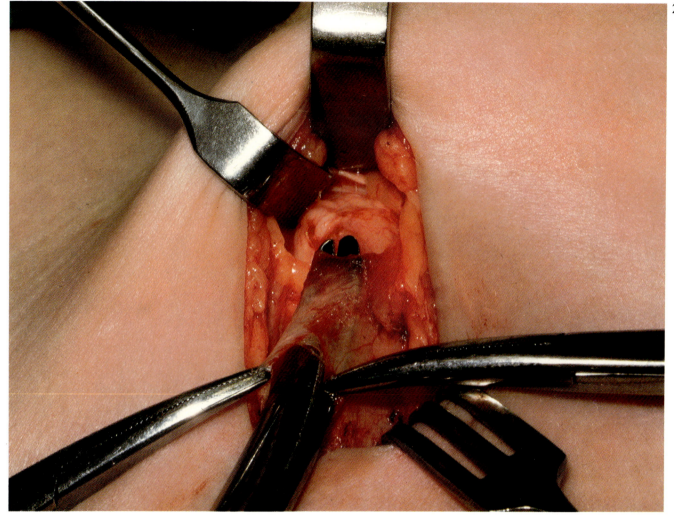

22 The anterior wall of the inguinal canal is opened by completing the division of the external oblique aponeurosis from the lateral opening through to the external inguinal ring. The location of the ileoinguinal nerve should again be checked before dividing the aponeurotic fibres.

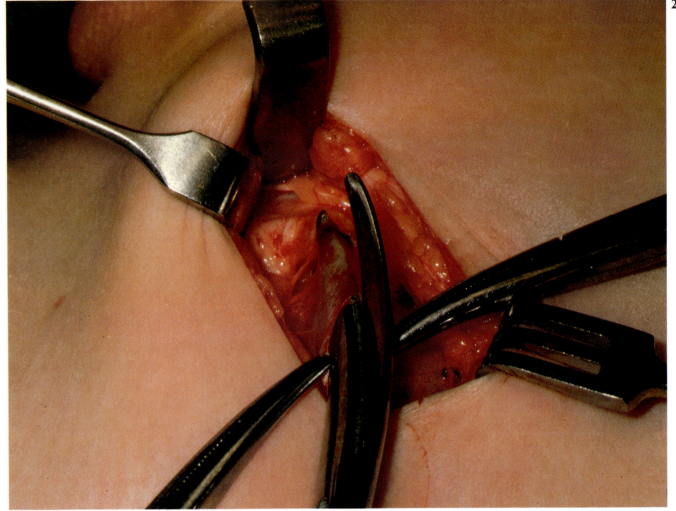

Mobilising spermatic cord and coverings

23 The spermatic cord and its coverings are gently lifted out of the inguinal canal using blunt dissecting forceps. The testis can be seen appearing at the medial end of the incision.

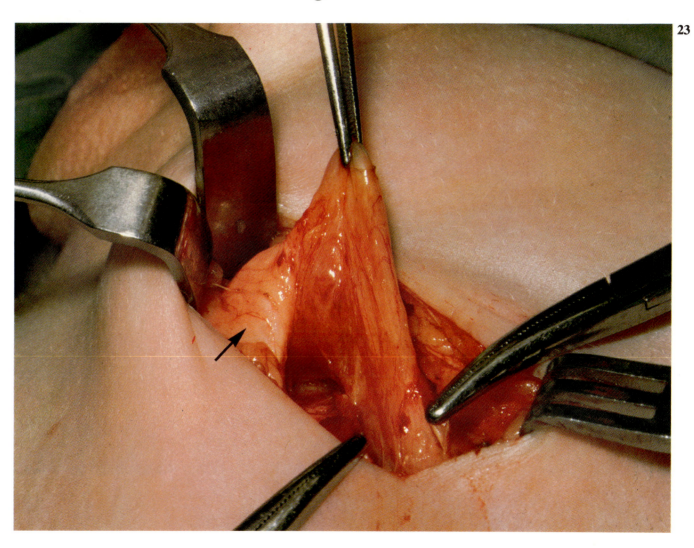

24   The spermatic cord is dissected off the floor of the inguinal canal. As the cord is elevated the small cremastic artery is seen passing from the inferior epigastric artery to supply the outer coverings of the cord. It is ligated and divided to avoid troublesome haemorrhage which may occur, should it be damaged at a later stage.

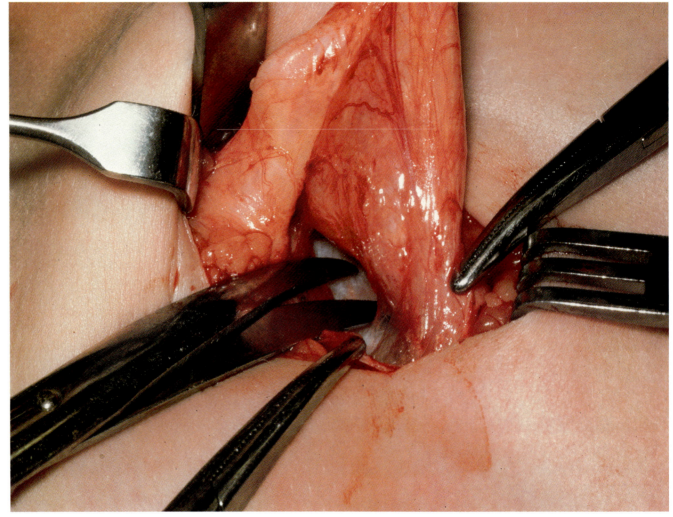

25 **The spermatic cord has been completely mobilised and attention is now directed towards the testis** which is carefully freed circumferentially leaving the inferior pole attached by the gubernaculum. This part of the procedure may be carried out using either blunt dissection with fine non-toothed dissecting forceps or by sharp dissection.

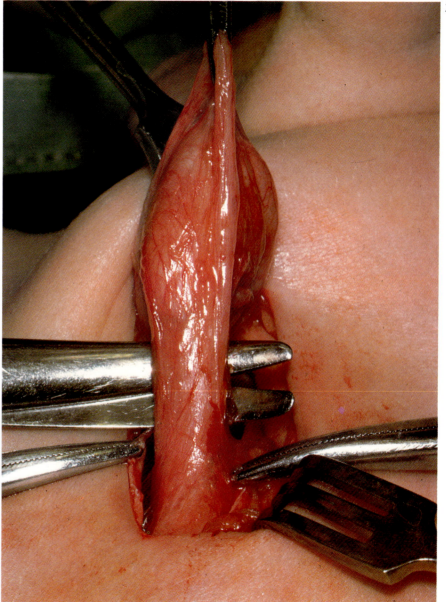

26 **The wide-based gubernaculum can be seen passing from the inferior pole of the testis towards the pubic tubercle.** Note the clean floor of the inguinal canal beneath the spermatic cord.

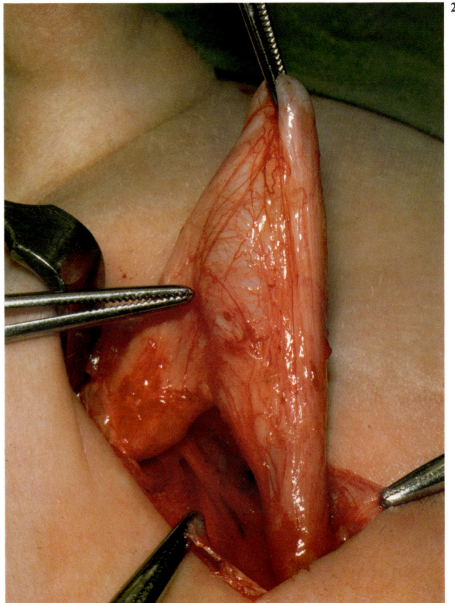

27

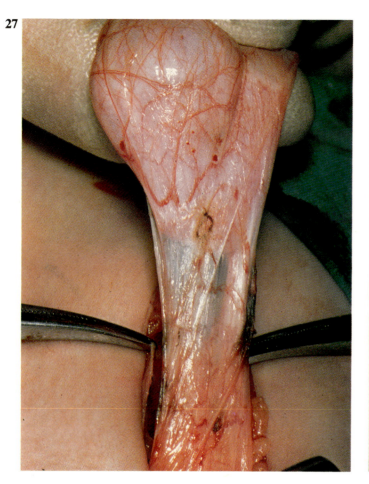

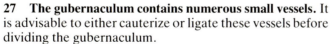

27   The gubernaculum contains numerous small vessels. It is advisable to either cauterize or ligate these vessels before dividing the gubernaculum.

Failure to attend to these vessels may result in a haematoma of the scrotum or of the inguinal wound.

28

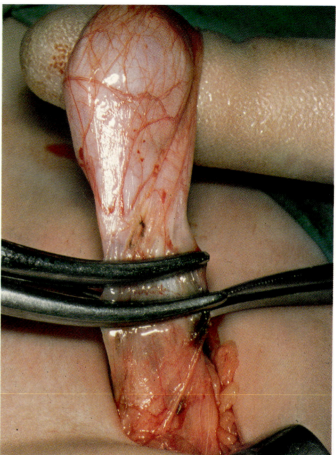

28   Artery clamps are applied to the gubernaculum well distal to the inferior pole of the testis. The vas deferens may loop down below the testis before joining the epididymis; it is imperative that the gubernaculum should not be clamped and divided before the precise position of the vas has been defined.

29 The gubernaculum has been divided and its distal end is ligated with 4.0 polyglycolic acid or chromic catgut ligature.

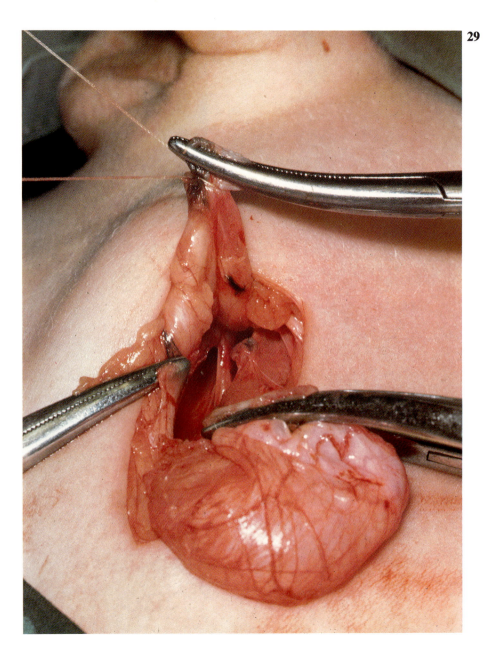

30 The proximal end of the gubernaculum is also ligated using the same material. The ligature is deliberately kept long and grasped in an artery forceps to assist with gentle traction during the separation of the cord structures.

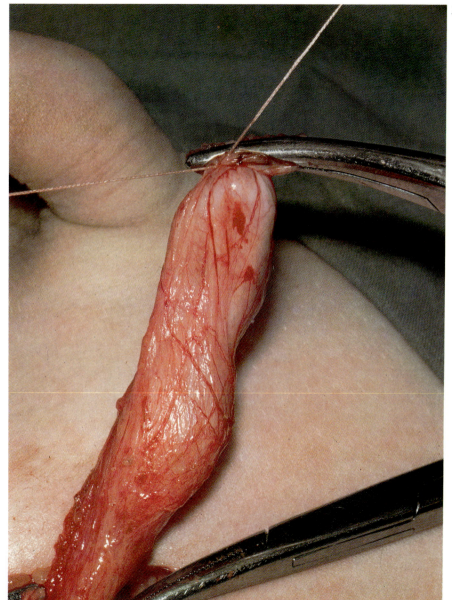

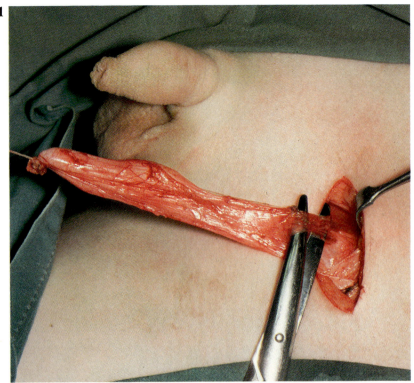

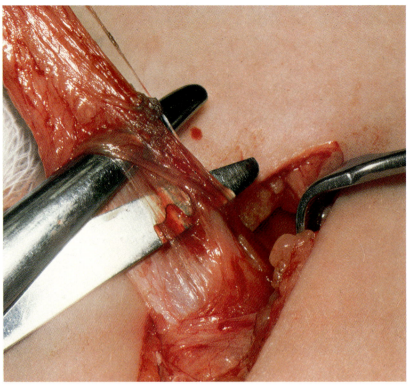

31   The fibres of the cremaster muscle, which arise from the internal oblique and transversus abdominus muscles and spiral around the cord towards the pubic tubercle, are dissected off the surface of the cord and divided.

32   A close-up view of the cremaster muscle fibres in the vicinity of the internal (deep) inguinal ring.

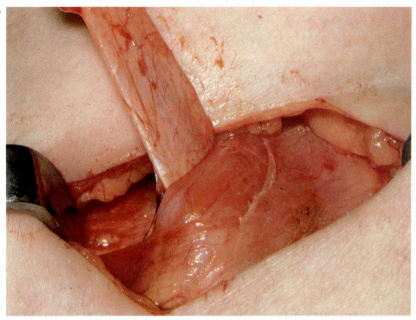

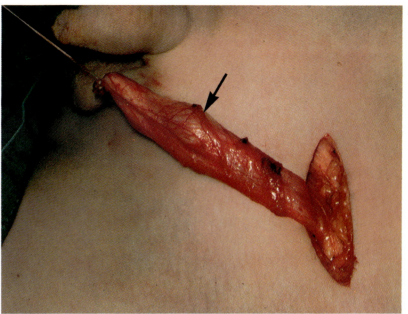

33 The spermatic cord has been completely cleared of cremaster muscle fibres and can be seen emerging from the internal inguinal ring. The ring lies just above the midpoint of the inguinal ligament and is bounded laterally by the angle between the transversus muscle fibres and the inguinal ligament.

34 The testis and spermatic cord have been completely mobilised up to the level of the internal ring. The ligature on the gubernaculum indicates that there is still a substantial distance between the testis and the left hemiscrotum.

Closure of the incomplete hernial sac

35 An indirect inguinal hernial sac (patent processus vaginalis) is present in all true incompletely descended testes and in 50 per cent of ectopic testes. The hernial sac in association with ectopic testes may be incomplete when it consists of a tongue-like projection of peritoneum overlying the anterior aspect of the spermatic cord. It descends only for approximately 1 cm onto the spermatic cord.

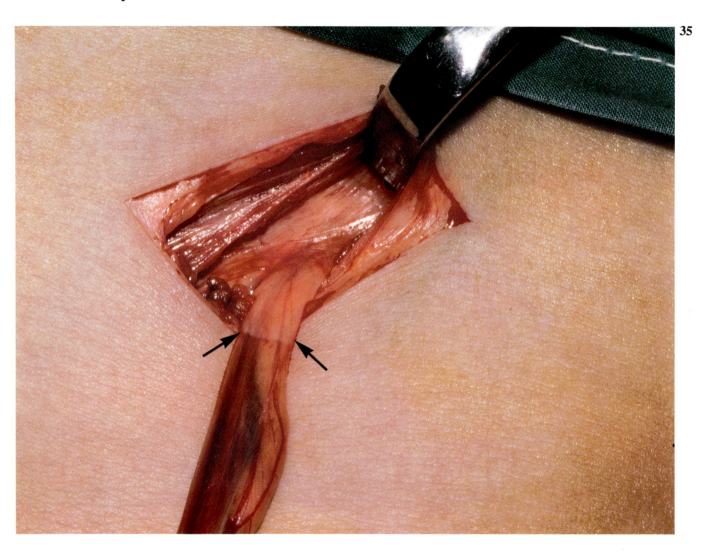

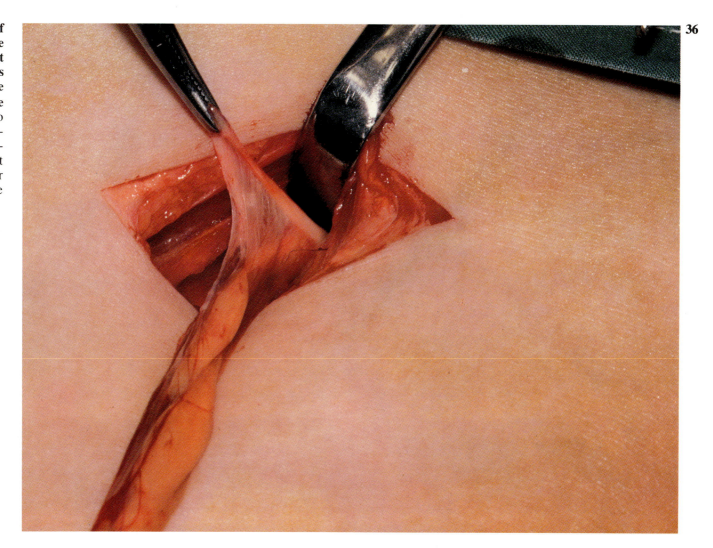

36 The projection of peritoneum forming the incomplete indirect inguinal hernial sac has been dissected off the anterior aspect of the spermatic any trauma to the underlying vas deferens or spermatic vessels. Further management of the hernial sac is similar to that of the complete hernial sac (see **54** to **57**).

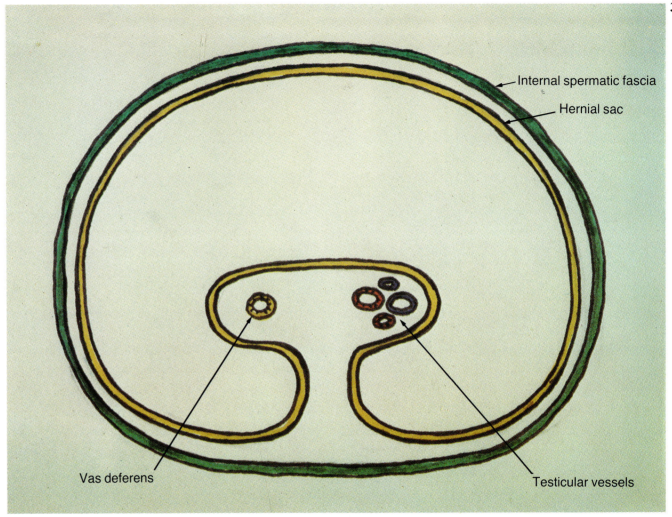

37 In the incompletely descended testis the indirect inguinal hernial sac is complete and surrounds the testis. The vas deferens and vessels invaginate into the hernial wall from the posterior surface and appear to be actually inside the hernial sac. By gently teasing apart the apposed walls on the posterior aspect of the hernial sac, using two fine non-toothed dissecting forceps, it is possible to isolate the vas and vessels without actually entering the sac. Some surgeons prefer to approach the sac from the anterior aspect. This inevitably leads to the sac being opened and requires a delicate and often difficult dissection of the posterior wall of the flimsy sac from the underlying vas and vessels.

Internal spermatic fascia

Hernial sac

Vas deferens

Testicular vessels

Identification of the complete hernial sac

38 The testis and spermatic cord are everted proximally over the anterior abdominal wall to expose the posterior surface of the spermatic cord. It is here that further dissection will take place to isolate the vas deferens and testicular vessels from the hernial sac.

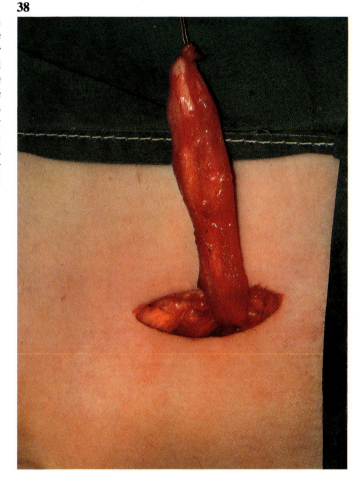

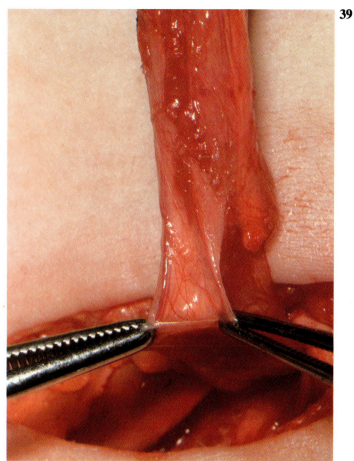

39 The two opposing surfaces of the hernial sac are gently teased apart posteriorly using fine blunt tissue forceps. This procedure is most conveniently performed mid-way between the testis and the internal (deep) inguinal ring. Should the hernial sac be inadvertently opened, the edges should be grasped with fine artery forceps and particular care taken that the complete circumference of the sac is isolated before ligating and dividing the sac at its neck.

Tears in the flimsy sac are prone to extend proximally creating difficulty in accurate closure of the orifice or neck of the hernia.

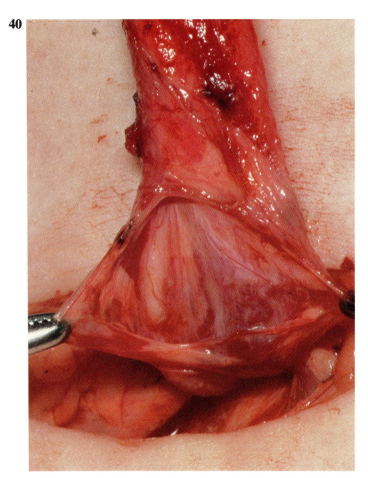

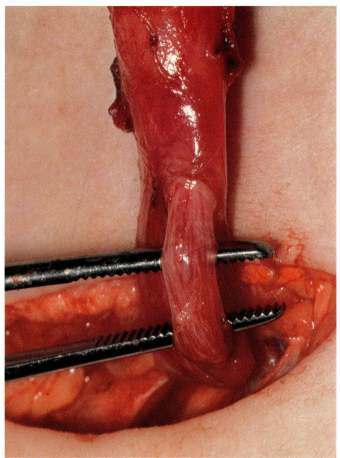

40 The apposed walls of the hernial sac have been separated posteriorly revealing the vas medially (on the left in the figure) and the testicular vessels laterally. The hernial sac has not been entered.

41 The testicular vessels are carefully separated from the underlying hernial sac. The vessels should not be grasped in the dissecting forceps but rather swept aside using the forceps. This is easily achieved once the correct plane of tissues has been entered.

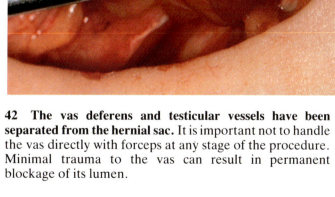

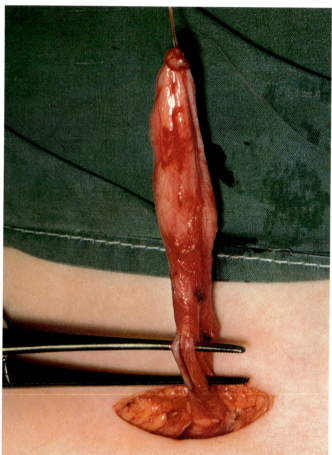

42 The vas deferens and testicular vessels have been separated from the hernial sac. It is important not to handle the vas directly with forceps at any stage of the procedure. Minimal trauma to the vas can result in permanent blockage of its lumen.

43 Full view of the operative site showing the vas and vessels separate from the hernial sac. The testis is completely surrounded by the patent processus vaginalis.

Spermatic cord returned to correct orientation

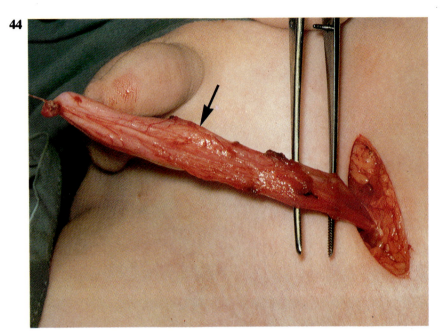

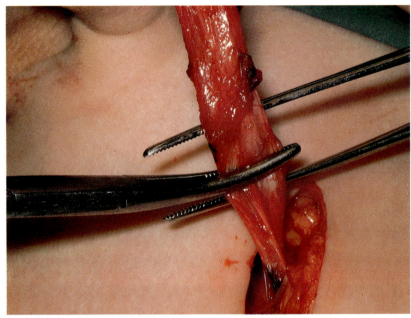

44   The spermatic cord is returned to its correct orientation by drawing the ligature on the gubernaculum down from the anterior abdominal wall towards the scrotum. The hernial sac now lies in its correct anatomical position in front of the vas and vessels. The testis is still well above the scrotum and further mobilisation of the testicular vessels is required.

45   An artery forceps is placed across the hernial sac. The position of the vas and vessels is checked to ensure that they are not included in the jaws of the forceps.

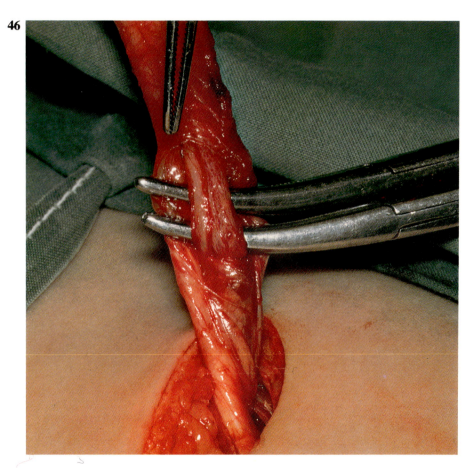

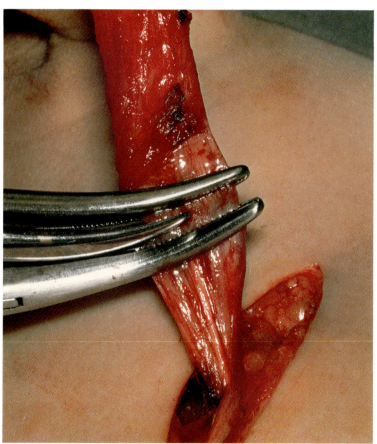

46   Posterior view of the vas and vessels with the two artery forceps across the hernial sac.

47   The hernial sac is divided between the artery forceps. The importance of identifying the position of the vas and vessels before clamping, ligating, or dividing any structure cannot be overemphasised.

Hernial sac divided

48 The hernial sac has been divided now. The vas and vessels are now all that maintain continuity with the testis.

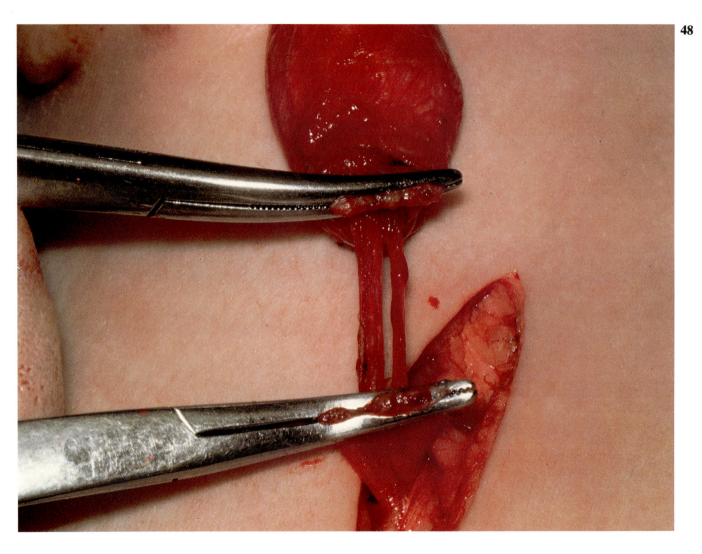

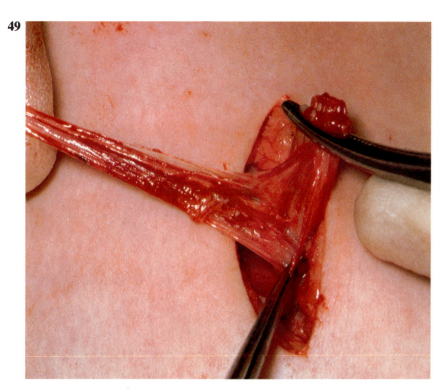

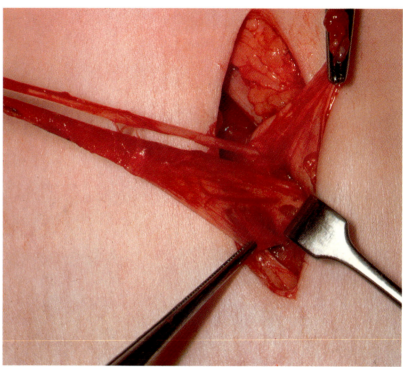

49   Attention is now directed to the lateral spermatic bands (Denis Browne). These bands in the retroperitoneal tissues extend from the testicular vessels to the lateral abdominal wall causing an acute angulation of the vessels. By dividing these bands as far proximally as possible, the course of the vessels is straightened thereby increasing the length of the 'spermatic cord'.

50   A further view of the lateral spermatic bands. The retractor is lifting the peritoneum forwards exposing the bands in the retroperitoneal tissues.

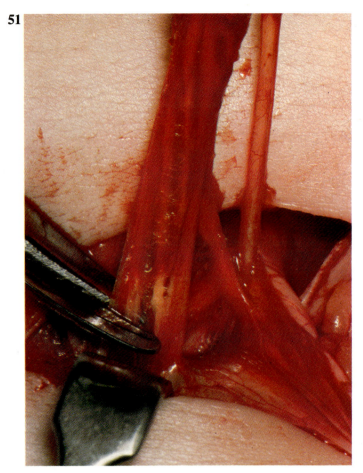

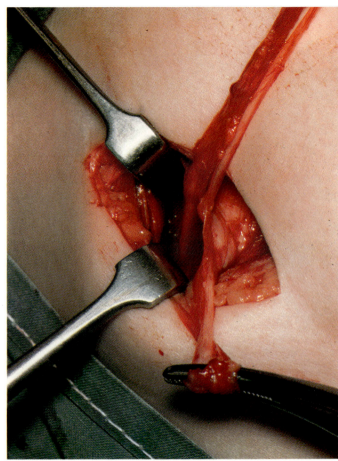

51   Division of the lateral spermatic bands is achieved by a combination of sharp and blunt dissection. These bands consist of loose fibrous tissue so that haemorrhage will not occur as a consequence of their division.

52   Elevation of the proximal end of the divided hernial sac (still held in an artery forceps) is used to achieve additional exposure of the retroperitoneal space for mobilisation of the testicular vessels.

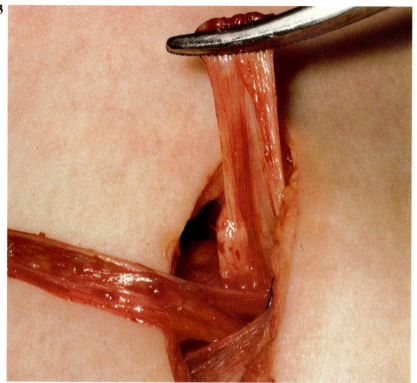

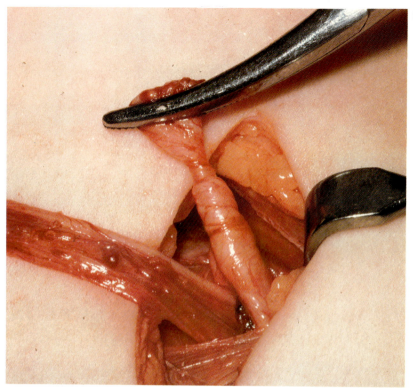

53 A close-up view at the internal inguinal ring showing the hernial sac held in an artery forceps and the vas and vessels disappearing proximally through the internal ring. Should additional exposure of the retroperitoneum be required, the fibres of internal and transversus muscles forming the lateral border of the internal ring may be divided.

54 The proximal end of the hernial sac is twisted a few times to ensure reduction of any contents and to facilitate accurate ligation of the neck of the sac.

Hernial sac transfixed and ligated

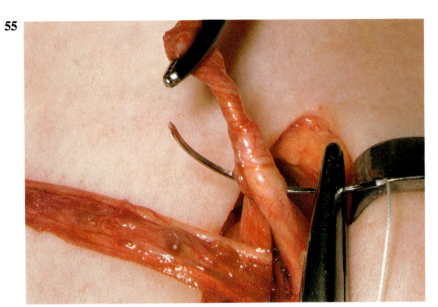

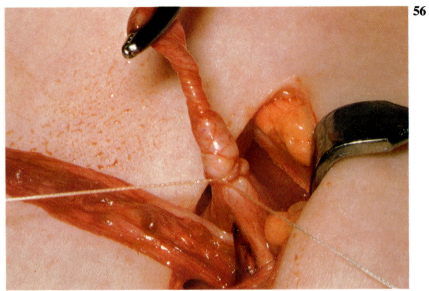

55 The hernial sac is transfixed and doubly ligated with 3.0 or 4.0 polyglycolic acid or silk suture. A slotted spoon (Denis Browne) may be used to prevent accidental trauma to the vas and vessels. The hernial sac is included in the slot of the spoon, while the vas and vessels are held posteriorly by the cup of the spoon.

56 The first ligature around the neck of the hernial sac is tied.

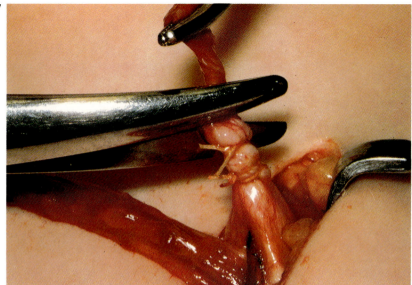

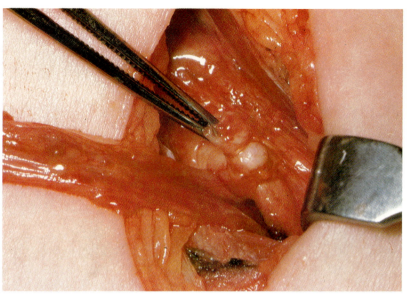

57 The second ligature around the neck of the hernial sac has been secured and the redundant part of the sac excised.

58 The medial border of the internal ring is formed by the inferior epigastric vessels. Where there is insufficient length of the testicular vessels, even after extensive retroperitoneal dissection, a few extra millimetres may be obtained by either ligating and dividing the inferior epigastric vessels, or by tunnelling the spermatic vessels and vas beneath these vessels.

59 A finger is inserted through the medial end of the groin incision to create a tunnel into the scrotum. The fibrous tissue preventing the testis from entering the scrotum is broken down by forcing the finger towards the scrotum until the tip of the finger reaches the most dependent part of the scrotal sac.

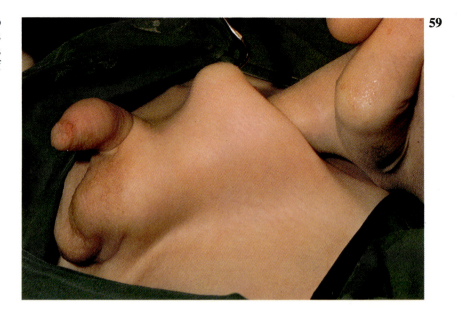

Fashioning of the dartos pouch

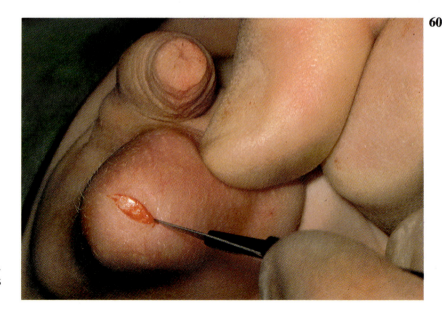

60 An incision is made through the skin at the base of the hemiscrotum. The incision extends through the skin and the closely adherent dartos muscle only.

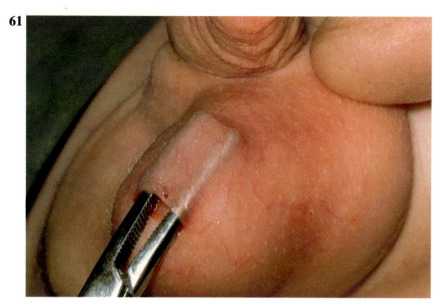

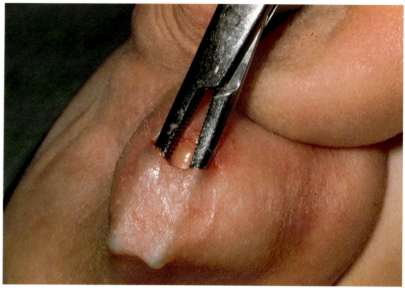

61 Using blunt dissection a pouch, large enough to accommodate the testis comfortably, is fashioned between the dartos muscle and the underlying loose fascia within the scrotum. If the pouch is too small, it will be difficult to place the testis in the pouch, and tension on the wound will predispose to dehiscence.

62 The subdartos pouch is now complete. Some authors advocate developing a pouch between the skin and the dartos muscle. This leaves a very thin layer of skin which is prone to slough. There are no advantages in placing the testis so superficial in the scrotum.

Reposition of the testis in the scrotum

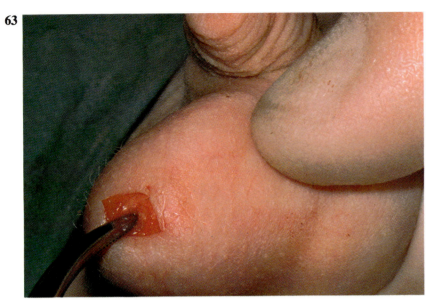

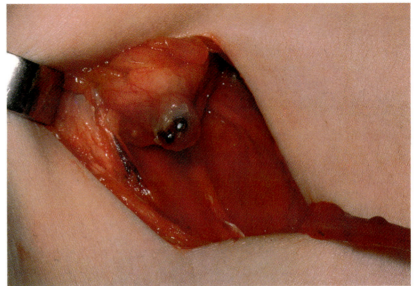

63 A long artery forceps is passed up from the scrotal incision to the groin using a finger inserted from above to guide it through the previously created tunnel.

64 The scrotal fascia is tented by the artery forceps and a small incision is made in this fascia to allow the tip of the forceps to appear in the groin wound. The incision should be large enough to allow the testis to be manipulated through but not so large that it will easily retract back into the groin.

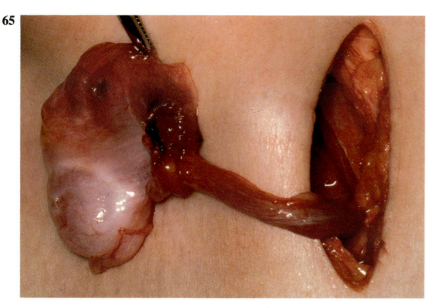

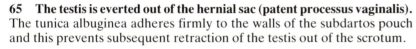

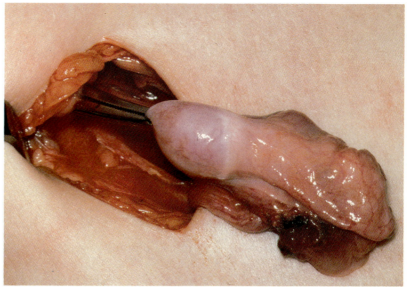

65   The testis is everted out of the hernial sac (patent processus vaginalis). The tunica albuginea adheres firmly to the walls of the subdartos pouch and this prevents subsequent retraction of the testis out of the scrotum.

66   The tunica albuginea of the testis is grasped in the artery forceps and the testis is pulled down into the scrotum. To avoid damage to the underlying testicular structures only the superficial layer of the tunica albuginea is included in the artery forceps.

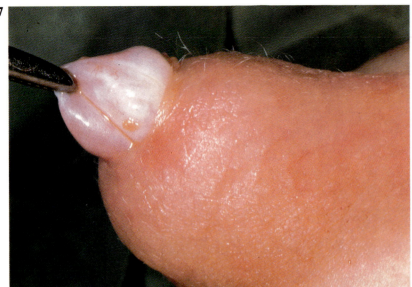

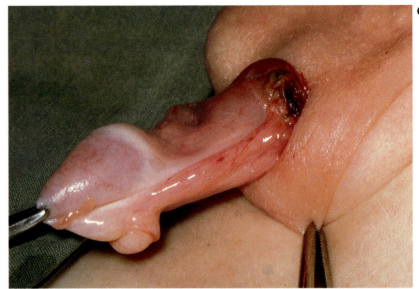

67   The testis is now pulled down into the scrotum after ensuring that the vas and vessels are correctly orientated and torsion of the cord has not occurred. The vas deferens always lies medial to the testicular vessels.

68   The testis is pulled out through the scrotal incision. The scrotal fascia is manipulated gently over the testis without enlarging the opening. A narrow opening will prevent retraction of the testis out of the scrotum. If the fascial orifice is considered too large (i.e. if the testis can be easily retracted back into the groin), it should be narrowed by inserting one or two sutures in the lateral angles.

69 **The testis is gently manipulated back into the dartos pouch.** This manoeuvre is facilitated by elevating the lateral edges of the scrotal incision with sharp skin hooks.

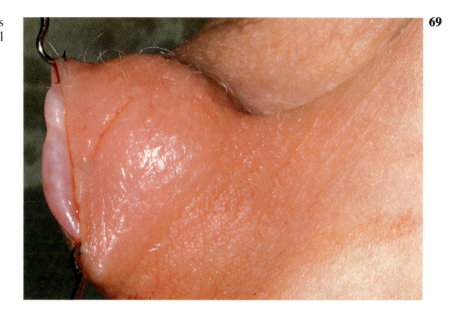

Closure of scrotal incision

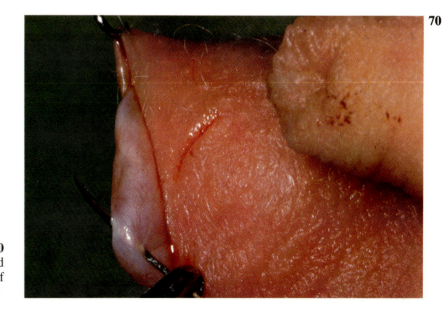

70 **The scrotal incision is closed with three inverting absorbable (5.0 chromic catgut or polyglycolic acid) sutures.** The middle suture is passed through the tunica albuginea of the testis to encourage firm adhesion of the testis to the dartos pouch.

Closure of inguinal incision

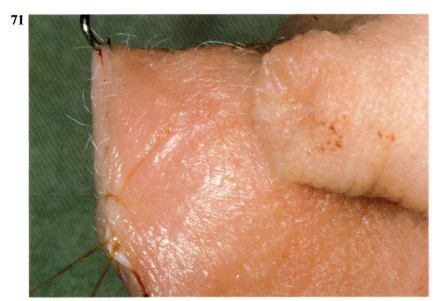

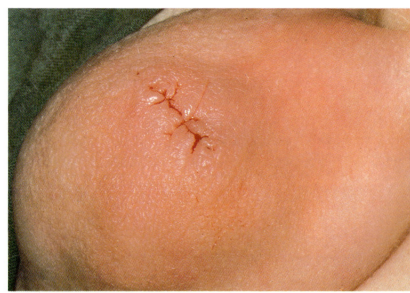

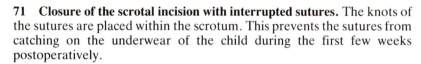

71 **Closure of the scrotal incision with interrupted sutures.** The knots of the sutures are placed within the scrotum. This prevents the sutures from catching on the underwear of the child during the first few weeks postoperatively.

72 **The scrotal incision has been completely closed.** Note the testis bulging in the dartos pouch in the most dependent part of the scrotum.

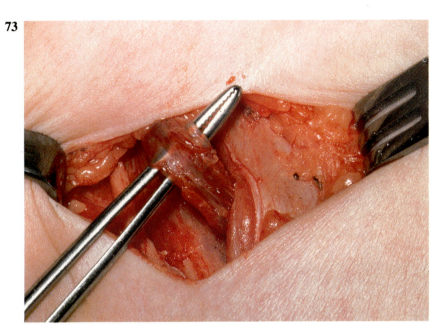

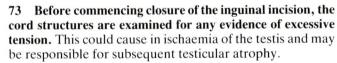

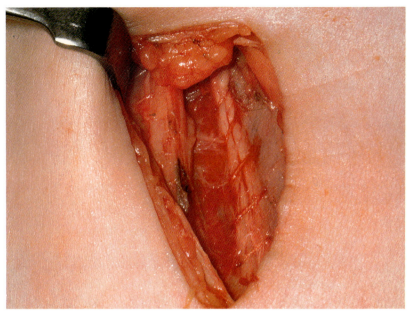

73 Before commencing closure of the inguinal incision, the cord structures are examined for any evidence of excessive tension. This could cause in ischaemia of the testis and may be responsible for subsequent testicular atrophy.

74 If division of the internal oblique muscle at the internal ring was necessary, these fibres should be re-approximated with interrupted sutures. Closure of the external oblique aponeurosis with 3.0 or 4.0 polyglycolic acid sutures should be carried out from lateral to medial.

Particular attention should be taken to avoid including the ileoinguinal nerve in the suture.

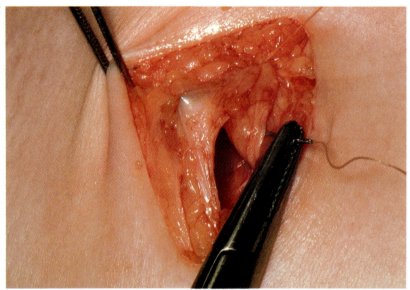

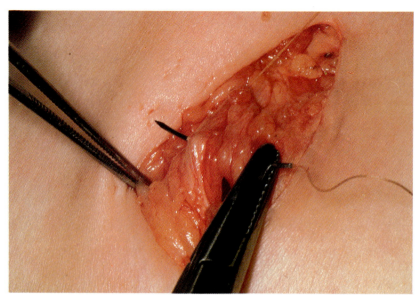

75 At the medial end sufficient external oblique aponeurosis should remain open to allow free passage for the vas and vessels through the reconstituted external (superficial) inguinal ring.

76 The fascia of Scarpa is closed as a separate layer with a continuous 4.0 polyglycolic acid suture.

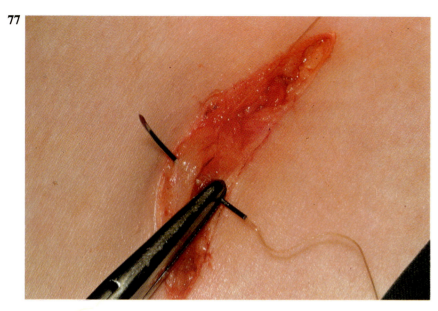

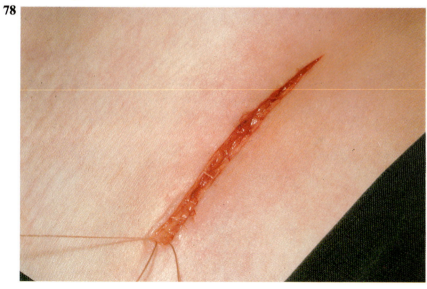

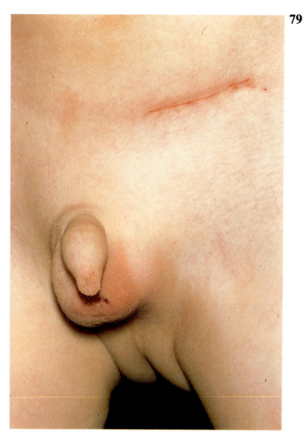

77 The subcutaneous fatty layer is closed as a separate layer with a few interrupted or a continuous 4.0 polyglycolic acid suture.

The separate closure of this layer eliminates tissue planes and avoids the possibility of fluid accumulating in the subcutaneous tissues. Such fluid collections may become infected with resultant abscess formation.

78 The skin of the inguinal incision is approximated with a continuous 4.0 polyglycolic acid or chromic catgut subcuticular suture.

79 Final appearance of the inguinal and scrotal incisions. The testis can be seen in the most dependent part of the scrotum. The subcuticular suture dispenses with the need to remove skin sutures.

Postoperative care

The patient may either be discharged from hospital on the evening after the orchidopexy (day-case) or on the first postoperative day. Prolonged hospitalisation and bed-rest are both unnecessary and costly. During the first few days after surgery the child will bend or crouch forwards while walking, but full recovery is remarkably rapid.

The position of the testis should be checked at two weeks and again six months postoperatively.

The parents and later the child should be instructed to report any subsequent swelling of either testis to their medical practitioner without delay.

Full activity and sport may be resumed within three to four weeks of the orchidopexy.

Complications are rare but may include the following:

i) Early: wound haematoma
                wound sepsis
                testicular necrosis
ii) Late: testicular retraction into the groin
                testicular atrophy
                malignancy

Further reading

Fonkalsrud, E.W. and Mengel, W., *The Undescended Testis*, Year Book Medical Publishing Inc., Chicago/London, 1981.

Scholtmeijer, R.J., Molenaar, J.C., Chadha, Dev R., Symposium on Undescended Testes, *European Journal of Pediatrics* (1982) **139**, 247-294.

Scorer, C.G. and Farrington, G.H., *Congenital Deformities of the Testis and Epididymis*, Butterworths, London, 1971.

Rajser, J. Symposium on Cryptorchidism,   *Urol. Clin. N. Amer.* (1982), Oct. 9,**3**, 313-442.

Index